Table of Contents

PREVIEW

Heart failure, sometimes known as congestive heart failure, occurs when your heart muscle doesn't pump blood as well as it should. Certain conditions, such as narrowed arteries in your heart (coronary artery disease) or high blood pressure, gradually leave your heart too weak or stiff to fill and pump efficiently.

HEART FAILURE DIET RECIPES

BREAKFAST

1. Pumpkin Apple Bread
Servings: 8 slices

Ingredients

- 2 cups all purpose flour
- 1 teaspoon baking soda
- 2 teaspoons cinnamon
- 2 teaspoons pumpkin spice *see post for suggestion
- 1 teaspoon table salt
- 2 large eggs
- 3/4 cup white sugar
- 1/2 cup light brown sugar
- 1 15oz can pumpkin puree (not pie filling)
- 1/2 cup vegetable or canola oil
- 1/4 cup apple juice
- 2/3 cup honeycrisp apples (about 1 apple), chopped small

Instructions

1. Adjust your oven rack to the lower 1/3rd of your oven. Preheat to 350°F degrees. Grease a 9x5 loaf pan well with extra oil. In one large bowl, combine the flour, baking soda, cinnamon, pumpkin spice, and salt and mix till combined.

2. In a small bowl, whisk the eggs and add white and brown sugar, mixing till combined. In another separate bowl, combine the pumpkin puree with oil and apple juice till smooth. Fold in the egg/sugar

mixture, then mix the wet ingredients into the dry ingredients. There will be a few lumps, this is ok. Finally add in the apples, stirring till just combined.

3. Pour the batter into the prepared loaf pan and bake uncovered for 30 minutes on the lower rack. Add a tented tin foil cover, so it gives the bread enough room to rise more. Bake another 30-35 minutes until a toothpick inserted in the center comes out almost clean. Allow it to cool 10-15 minutes before removing from the baking pan. It should slide right out if oiled correctly, but running a knife along the sides to loosen it may help.

2. Blackberry Muffins

Servings: 12 muffins

Ingredients

- 8 tablespoons (1/2 cup) unsalted butter, at room temperature
- 3 oz cream cheese, at room temperature
- 1/2 cup white sugar
- 2 large eggs
- 1 teaspoon vanilla extract
- 2 cups all purpose flour
- 2 teaspoons baking powder
- 1/2 teaspoon baking soda
- 1/2 teaspoon kosher salt
- 1/2 cup milk
- 1 1/2 cups fresh blackberries, chopped into smaller pieces (they will fall apart a bit)
- Optional: turbinado sugar for sprinkling on top

Instructions

1. Preheat oven to 375 degrees F. In a mixing bowl, combine room temperature butter (left out about 20-30 min), cream cheese, and sugar. With an electric mixer, beat on medium speed till smooth and combined. On low speed, add eggs one at a time until just combined. Add 1 teaspoon of vanilla.

2. In a separate mixing bowl, combine flour, baking powder, baking soda, and salt. Alternate adding flour and milk into the butter mixture while mixing on low speed till combined. Fold in chopped blackberries with a spatula.

3. Prepare a muffin tin with paper cups and spoon the mixture into each cup, filling to the top. Add a pinch of turbinado sugar to the tops (if using for extra crunch). Bake for 23-25 minutes, until light brown on top and a toothpick inserted in the center comes out clean. (If using frozen blackberries, you may need to bake a few minutes longer)
4. Leave the muffins in the tin for 3-5 minutes and then remove to a cooling rack.

3. Cinnamon Oat Scones

Prep Time:30 minutes
Cook Time: 14 minutes
Total Time: 1 hr 15 minutes
Servings: 8 scones

Ingredients

- 2 cups all purpose flour *Use 1:1 gluten free
- 1/4 cup oat flour
- 1 tablespoon aluminum free baking powder
- 1/4 teaspoon baking soda
- 1/3 cup white sugar
- 1/2 teaspoon salt
- 6 tablespoons chilled shortening
- 1/3 cup oat milk
- 2 teaspoons distilled white vinegar
- 1 cold large egg
- 1 tablespoon vanilla extract

Cinnamon Sugar Topping
- 1/3 cup shortening
- 1 tablespoon honey
- 1/4 cup brown sugar
- 1/4 cup turbinado sugar
- 1/2 cup oat flour
- 1 teaspoon cinnamon
- 1/2 cup rolled oats
- 1/8 teaspoon salt

Instructions

1. Cover a sheet pan with parchment paper or a nonstick mat. In a large bowl, stir together the all

purpose (GF) flour, oat flour, baking powder, baking soda, sugar, and salt. Add in the cold shortening and using a pastry cutter or clean hands, combine the shortening into the flour mixture until crumbly.

2. In a medium bowl, whisk together the oat milk, white vinegar, egg, and vanilla extract. Pour this into the dry mixture, and stir with a wooden spoon until a dough forms. If the dough appears too dry, you can add a little more oat milk.

3. Lightly sprinkle some additional flour over the prepared sheet pan. Place the dough onto the prepared pan, and form into a disc. Don't overwork the dough here, but you can sprinkle on more flour if the dough is too sticky to work with. You want the disc to be about 1 1/2 inches thick. Set aside.

4. In a medium bowl, stir together the shortening, honey, brown sugar, turbinado sugar, oat flour, cinnamon, oats, and salt. Using a fork or your hands, work in the shortening until crumbs form. Be sure to mix this thoroughly so there's no big lumps of shortening. Pile the crumb topping on top of the scone dough. Press it evenly into the disc, reaching the edges, and creating a fairly even layer. This will make your dough disc a bit thinner- about 1 inch thick. Cover the dough disk with plastic wrap, and chill for 30 minutes.

5. While the dough is chilling, preheat your oven to 425 degrees F, and prepare a second pan with parchment paper. Remove the dough from the fridge, and use a knife or bench scrapper to cut the disc into 8 even triangles. Place onto your

parchment lined sheet pan, leaving an inch or two between each scone.

6. Bake for 14-17 minutes, or until the scones are puffed and golden brown on the edges and top. Let the scones cool on the sheet pan for about 5 minutes, and then use a spatula to move them to a cooling rack. The topping will have bubbled over the sides of the scones- and that's ok!

4. Strawberry Cream Cheese Muffins

Prep Time: 15 minutes

Cook Time: 25 minutes

Total Time: 40 minutes

Servings: 12 muffins

Ingredients

- 8 tablespoons (1/2 cup) unsalted butter, at room temperature
- 1/2 cup sugar
- 2 large eggs
- 3 oz cream cheese (block style, not tub)
- 1 teaspoon vanilla extract
- 2 cups all purpose flour
- 2 teaspoons baking powder
- 1/2 teaspoon baking soda
- 1/2 teaspoon kosher salt
- 1/2 cup milk
- 2 cups fresh strawberries, cut into small pieces

Instructions

1. Preheat oven to 375 degrees F. In a large bowl, combine room temperature butter (left out about 20-30 min, not melted), cream cheese, and sugar. With an electric mixer on medium speed, beat until it's nicely combined and smooth. On low speed, add in eggs until just combined along with 1 teaspoon of vanilla.

2. In a separate bowl, mix flour with baking powder, baking soda, and salt until combined. Alternate adding flour mixture to the butter/cream cheese mixture with the milk on low speed until just combined. Stir in the fresh strawberry pieces by hand with a spatula.

3. Prepare a non stick baking sheet (or add paper cups) and spoon the mixture into each cup until full and evenly dispersed. It should fill almost to the top. If you'd like, you can use a little extra sugar on top to provide a bit of a crunch. Bake for approximately 25-30 minutes until cooked through and light brown on top. A toothpick inserted in the center should come out almost clean.

4. Remove from the pan and cool on a wire rack. See post for instructions on freez.

5. Strawberry Bread

Prep Time: 10 minutes

Cook Time: 1 hr

Total Time : 1 hrs 10 minutes

Servings: 12 people

Ingredients

- 1/2 cup (4oz) softened, unsalted butter
- 3/4 cup organic cane sugar
- 3 oz cream cheese
- 2 eggs
- 1 tsp vanilla extract
- 1 cup organic oat flour
- 1 cup brown rice flour
- 1/2 tsp sea salt
- 2 tsp baking powder
- 1/2 tsp baking soda
- 1/2 cup whole milk
- 2 cups washed, strawberries cut into small pieces

Instructions

1. Take your butter out of the fridge about an hour or so before starting the recipe. Room temperature butter is much easier to work with.

2. Preheat oven to 350. With electric mixer cream butter, sugar, cream cheese, eggs and vanilla until fluffy. Mix in the flour, baking powder, baking soda

and salt. Blend flour mixture with butter mixture just until blended.

3. Add milk and only stir just enough to blend -- do not over stir. Carefully just fold in cut strawberries. Dough mixture will be thick.

4. Grease a 9x5 inch loaf pan. (Tip...I always use the butter wrapper of the stick of butter I used above. There's plenty of residual butter there for greasing.)

5. Bake in a 350 degree oven for 60 minutes. Cool before serving.

6. Quiche Florentine

Prep Time: 15 minutes

Cook Time: 50 minutes

Total Time: 1 hrs 5 minutes

Servings: 4 people

Ingredients

- 1 9" frozen pie crust
- 3 large eggs
- 3/4 cup whole milk
- 1/4 cup heavy cream
- 3 oz chevre (soft goat cheese)
- 1/2 cup loosely chopped fresh spinach
- 1 shallot, chopped
- 1/4-1/2 teaspoon kosher salt and black pepper
- fresh thyme (optional)

Instructions

1. Remove pie crust from freezer and allow it to warm while you preheat your oven. When softened a bit, poke holes all around the crust with the tines of a fork. If you want your crust to not puff up even more, fill it with pie weights or beans. Pre-bake your pie crust according to package directions (mine was 425 degrees F for 15-20 minutes) on the bottom 1/3rd of your oven, until very lightly browned.

2. Meanwhile, mix together the eggs, milk, cream and whisk till combined. Then add goat cheese (crumble

with your fingers), spinach, and chopped shallot with kosher salt and black pepper and stir. The goat cheese will not fully combine, but that's ok, it will melt down.

3. Remove pre-baked pie crust from the oven, change the temperature to 400 degrees F, and pour in the filling. It's really ok if you pie bottom breaks a part a bit, you won't be able to tell once it's baked.

4. Bake at 400 degrees F for about 50 minutes, until the center is puffed up. It should have just a slight jiggle, not a wave, when you move it around. Allow it to set/cool for about 5-10 minutes before eating. I LOVE a little fresh thyme leaves on top if you have them on hand.

7. Buckwheat Pancakes with Bananas

Serves: 2

Ingredients

- 1 cup buckwheat flour
- 1 Tbsp brown sugar
- 2 Tbsp potato starch
- 1/2 tsp salt
- 1 tsp baking powder
- 1 cup rice milk
- 2 Tbsp canola oil
- Vegetable cooking spray, for frying
- 2 large bananas, sliced
- Brown rice syrup, to serve

Instructions

1. Combine dry ingredients in a medium bowl. Add rice milk and canola oil, and whisk until well combined. If batter seems very thick, you may want add a little extra rice milk or water.

2. Preheat a large nonstick skillet over medium heat. Spray with vegetable cooking spray.

3. With a ladle, pour batter to the size you prefer. Even out batter on skillet with back of a spoon. Cook pancake on medium high heat for a few minutes until bubbles appear. Flip over and continue frying until cooked (a properly cooked pancake appears dense and not sticky when cut in the middle).

4. Repeat previous step until batter is gone.

5. Serve pancakes with banana slices and brown rice syrup.

8. Fantastic Fiber Muffins
Ingredients

- 1 1/2 cups wheat bran
- 1 cup nonfat milk (or milk substitute)
- 1/2 cup unsweetened applesauce
- 1 egg
- 2/3 cup brown sugar
- 1/2 cup all-purpose flour
- 1/2 cup whole wheat flour
- 1 tsp baking powder
- 1 tsp baking soda
- 1/2 tsp salt
- 1 cup organic apples, washed, cored, chopped

Instructions

1. Preheat oven to 375°F (190°C, gas mark 5).

2. Combine wheat bran and milk, and let stand for 15 minutes.

3. In a large bowl, whisk together apple sauce, egg, and brown sugar. Stir in bran mixture and mix well.

4. In a small bowl, combine all-purpose flour, whole wheat flour, baking powder, baking soda, and salt. Stir into bran mixture and mix until just blended (do not over-mix). Fold in chopped apples.

5. Fill prepared muffin cups with batter (about two thirds full). Bake for about 15-20 minutes.

9. Gluten-Free Carrot Muffins

Yields: Servings 12

Ingredients

- 1 egg
- 1 cup rice milk
- 4 tbsp canola oil
- 2 cups quinoa flour or other gluten-free flour
- 1 tsp guar gum
- 1 tbsp flaxseed meal
- 3 1/2 tsp gluten-free baking powder
- 1/2 tsp salt
- 1 tsp cinnamon
- 1/4 cup brown sugar
- 1 cup organic carrots, grated

Instructions
1. Preheat oven to 400 degrees F (200 degrees C, gas mark 6)

2. Beat together egg, rice milk, and canola oil. Combine dry ingredients in a separate bowl.

3. Add liquid ingredients to dry ingredients and mix until just blended (do not over-mix). Fold in grated carrots and raisins.

4. Fill 12 paper muffin cups with batter (about two thirds full). Bake for 20 minutes.

10. Fully Stuffed Sweet Potatoes

Ingredients

- 2 medium sweet potatoes
- 1 tsp cumin
- ¼ tsp coriander
- ¼ tsp salt
- freshly ground black pepper
- 1 medium tomato, diced small
- 2 scallions, finely sliced
- ¾ cup black beans
- ½ lime, juiced
- 1 Tbsp freshly minced cilantro for garnish

Instructions

1. Preheat the oven to 450F.
2. Wash, scrub and dry the sweet potatoes.
3. Place a drying rack on top of a cookie sheet and put the sweet potatoes on top. By baking on a rack, no part of the skin will get soggy which will make stuffing them easier. Bake for approximately an hour turning every 20 minutes. (The sweet potatoes are done when they are soft to the touch and just starting to puff up, so you can tell the flesh is shifting away from the skin.)

4. Remove from the oven and let cool enough to handle, about 15 minutes.

5. Using a sharp knife gently slice away the top third of the sweet potato. With a small spoon carefully scoop away the inside of the sweet potato and put the flesh into a medium bowl.

6. Mash the flesh with a fork and whip in cumin, coriander, salt and a generous amount of freshly ground pepper. Stir in tomatoes, scallions, black beans and lime juice.

7. Divide the mixture in half and carefully stuff back into the potato skins, you can overfill them as long as they can stay upright.

8. Place potatoes back on the rack and bake for another 15 minutes.

9. Serve hot garnished with cilantro.

11. Warm Lentil Salad

Servings: 4

Ingredients

- 1 cup brown lentils
- 1 large orange carrot
- 1 large parsnip
- 2 large purple carrots
- 1 large leek
- 3 cups arugula lightly packed
- 2 tablespoons lemon juice from one fresh lemon
- 2 tablespoons honey
- 2 tablespoons olive oil plus extra to toss with vegetables
- 2 sprigs fresh thyme
- salt and pepper

Instructions

1. Preheat oven to 375 degrees and spray a baking pan with nonstick cooking spray.

2. Simmer lentils in 2 cups of water and 1/2 teaspoon of salt if desired, for 20-30 minutes or until tender. Drain any remaining water and let lentils cool a bit.

3. Peel carrots and parsnip and cut into 1/2 inch wide coins. Toss with up to 1 tablespoon of olive oil and sprinkle with salt and pepper. Spread vegetables in

one layer on the baking sheet. Reserve any remaining oil in the bowl for the leeks. Roast vegetables for about 15-20 minutes or until tender, flipping them halfway through so they caramelize evenly.

4. Trim leak, cutting off bulb and dark green stems, and any tough outer layer of the light green stems. If desired, reserve bulb and dark stems for stock.
5. Slice light green part into thin round strips, and rinse well to remove any dirt or sand. Place leeks in the bowl and toss with the oil, salt and pepper that remains from the vegetables.

6. When the vegetables are tender, remove from the oven and toss with the lentils in a large mixing bowl.

7. Spread the leeks on the baking pan, and roast for 10-12 minutes until they caramelize and start to turn dark and crispy.

8. Meanwhile, prepare the vinaigrette: Mix lemon juice, honey and 2 tablespoons olive oil together. Remove thyme leaves from their stem and add to vinaigrette. Season with salt and pepper.

9. Pour dressing over vegetables and lentils, toss to combine.

10. Serve lentil-vegetables over a bed of arugula, and sprinkle with crisped leeks.

12. Quinoa and Lentil Power Bowl

Ingredients

For the squash:

- 2 cups butternut squash, cubed
- 1/2 tablespoon extra virgin olive oil
- 1/2 teaspoon chili powder
- Salt and pepper, to taste
- For the quinoa and lentils:
- 2 cups vegetable stock, divided
- 1/3 cup lentils, uncooked
- 1/3 cup dry quinoa
- For the greens:
- 1 teaspoon extra virgin olive oil
- 1 garlic clove, chopped
- 4 cups kale (or other dark leafy green)
- Salt and pepper, to taste

For the eggs:

- 2 eggs

Instructions

1. Preheat oven to 400°F. On a lined baking sheet, gently toss squash in olive oil, chili powder, salt and pepper until coated.

2. Roast for 30-35 minutes, tossing halfway through, until soft to fork. Remove from oven and divide in serving bowls. Alternatively, you can use leftover or pre-prepared cooked squash.

3. While squash is cooking, prepare lentils according to package instructions, using 1 cup vegetable stock in place of water. Do not salt the stock. Set aside.

4. In another saucepan, prepare quinoa. Add quinoa to saucepan with 1 cup vegetable stock (add a pinch of salt if your stock is unsalted). Bring to a boil, then cover and reduce to a simmer and cook for 9 minutes. Turn off the heat, but leave saucepan covered for at least 10 minutes.

5. When both lentils and quinoa are done cooking, combine in a bowl, then divide among serving bowls.

6. In the meantime, coat a medium-sized sauté pan with 1/2 tablespoon olive oil. Gently sauté garlic in olive oil, then add greens. Cook until greens are wilted, but not soggy. Add to serving bowls.

7. Using the same pan as the greens, prepare your fried egg. Cooking one at a time, crack egg carefully onto pan. Cook until white becomes nearly opaque, about 1 minute. Carefully flip and cook for another 30 seconds. Yolk should still be runny when done. Place atop rest of ingredients in the bowl. Repeat with the second egg.

8. To assemble bowls, divide ingredients and arrange in bowls, as desired. Top with egg. Sprinkle with additional freshly ground black pepper (and hot sauce, if desired). Enjoy!

13. Grilled Veggie Nourish Bowl

Prep Time: 15 minutes

Cook Time: 15 minutes

Total Time: 30 minutes

Servings: 4 servings

Ingredients

- 2 tablespoons olive oil
- 1/4 teaspoon sea salt
- 1/4 teaspoon black pepper
- 2 large zucchini, sliced 1/4" thick
- 2 medium yellow squash, sliced 1/4" thick
- 2 cups grape tomatoes
- 1 (15 ounce) can chickpeas, drained and rinsed well
- 3 tablespoons shelled hemp seeds
- 1 1/2 cups whole grain sorghum, cooked

Tahini Dressing:

- 1/3 cup tahini
- 1 clove garlic, minced
- 1/4 teaspoon ground ginger
- 2 tablespoons lemon juice
- 1 tablespoon sorghum syrup, or maple syrup
- 1/4 cup + 1 tablespoon water

Instructions

1. Prepare grill on medium to medium-low heat. Using
   ½ teaspoon olive oil, lightly grease grill grate with a
   wire-bristled brush.

2. In a large plastic resealable bag, place sliced zucchini,
   yellow squash, remaining olive oil, sea salt, and
   pepper. Seal bag and shake well to coat the zucchini
   and yellow squash.

Stack grape tomatoes on skewers.

1. Grill the zucchini, yellow squash, and tomatoes for 3
   minutes, flip vegetables and grill an additional 3-4
   minutes or until tender and lightly browned (grape
   tomatoes may cook faster than other vegetables.)
   Remove from heat and set vegetables aside.

2. In a small bowl prepare dressing – add Tahini, garlic,
   ginger, lemon juice and sorghum syrup, mix together
   well. Add water and whisk until emulsified.

3. In 4 bowls, evenly distribute sorghum to the bottom of
   the bowl and top with grilled zucchini, yellow squash,
   tomatoes, chickpeas, and hemp hearts. Drizzle 2
   tablespoons of the Tahini dressing over vegetables

14. Winter Godess Bowl with Quinoa and Avocado Citrus Dressing

Ingredients

- 1/4 cup quinoa (Used the packet of Trader Joe's fully cooked organic quinoa (frozen section)
    - 3-4 slices of Chiogga beets
- 2 eggs hard boiled or soft boiled (made mine in the Instant Pot on steam for 4 minutes)
  3-4 red chard leaves, steamed
- For the sautéed squash and apples:
- 1/2 gala apple, diced
- 1 cup butternut squash, diced
- 1 small red onion, diced
- 2 Tbsp. of EVOO (extra virgin olive oil)
- salt, pepper and red pepper to taste
- For the avocado citrus dressing (makes a large batch, use about 2 Tbsp. for the bowl):
- 2 avocados
- juice of 1 Meyer lemon
- 2 cloves garlic
- 1/4 cup olive oil
- 1-2 Tbsp. apple cider vinegar
- 1 Tbsp. grainy mustard
- salt and pepper to taste

Instructions

Microwave or cook the quinoa and slightly steam the red chard. Once done, set aside. Cook the soft to hard boiled eggs and let sit in a ice water bath. Once cooled, remove shell and set aside.

1. On medium heat, place 2 Tbsp. of olive oil in a non-stick pan and add the apples, butternut squash, and onion to sauté. Add the salt, pepper, and red pepper to taste. Cook down until just slightly soft (about 10 minutes).
2. Next, in a VitaMix or very good blender, add all the ingredients for the sauce and blend until smooth. Place in a bowl.

3. Final step: Assemble. Place the red chard leaves at the bottom of the bowl, add 1/2 cup quinoa, 1/2 cup apples and butternut squash, beet slices, 1 or 2 eggs, and dress with 2 Tbsp. of the avocado citrus dressing.

15. Chicken Shawarma

Prep Time: 15 Minutes

Cook Time: 15 Minutes

Total Time: 30 Minutes

Servings: 4

Ingredients

- 1 1/2 pounds boneless skinless chicken thighs
- 4 tablespoons lemon juice
- 4 tablespoons extra virgin olive oil
- 4 cloves garlic minced
- 2 teaspoons ground cumin
- 2 teaspoons paprika
- 1 teaspoon turmeric
- 1/2 teaspoon ground cinnamon
- 1 teaspoon salt
- 1 teaspoon pepper
- chopped fresh parsley for serving if desired

Instructions

1. Add chicken to a large ziplock bag along with all of the ingredients except the chopped fresh parsley.

2. Cover and store in the refrigerator for at least 1 hour or overnight.

3. When you are ready to cook preheat oven to 425 F degrees.

4. Place chicken in a greased baking dish and bake until golden brown and cooked through.

(Mine took about 15 minutes because the chicken was on the thinner side).

5. In the last minute or two of cooking switch the oven to Broil. Cook chicken for 1-2 minutes until golden brown and crispy.

6. Remove from the oven and allow the chicken to rest for a couple of minutes before slicing.

7. Top with chopped fresh parsley if desired.

8. Serve the chicken in a pita or on top of a salad or over rice!

16. Greek Healthy Meal Prep

Prep Time 30 minutes

Cook Time 30 minutes

Total Time 1 hour

Servings: 5

Ingredients

Greek-Seasoned Chicken
- 3 medium boneless skinless chicken breasts
- 1 tablespoon extra virgin olive oil
- 1 teaspoons dried oregano
- 1/2 teaspoon dried thyme
- 1/2 teaspoon dried basil
- 1/2 teaspoon dried minced onion
- 1/2 teaspoon garlic powder
- 1 teaspoon salt

Tzatziki
- 1/2 large cucumber, unpeeled and grated
- 1 cup plain full-fat Greek yogurt or coconut yogurt
- 2 large garlic cloves, finely minced
- 2 Tablespoons extra virgin olive oil
- 1 Tablespoon white vinegar
- 1/2 teaspoon salt
- 1 Tablespoon minced fresh dill

Cauliflower Tabbouleh
- 1 bag bag of cauliflower rice, thawed
- 1/2 medium cucumber, unpeeled and diced
- 1 cup tomatoes, diced (about 2 Roma)

- 1 1/2 cups flat-leaf parsley, chopped
- 1/4 cup mint leaves, chopped (optional_
- 2 scallions, white and pale-green parts only, sliced thin
- 1 garlic clove, minced fine
- 2 tablespoons extra-virgin olive oil, divided
- 1/4 teaspoon finely grated lemon zest
- 2 tablespoons fresh lemon juice
- 1/4 teaspoon crushed red pepper flakes
- 1 teaspoon salt, plus more to taste

- Greek Meal Prep Bowls
- 3 tbsp hummus or baba ganoush, about 2-3 tablespoons per bowl (about 3/4 cup total)
- 5 kalamata olives, about 5 per bowl
- crumbled feta, if desired

Instructions

Tzatziki:

1. Place grated cucumber (for tzatziki) on a paper towel and gather edges together. Gently squeeze the bundle to get rid of as much liquid as possible, then place on top of a sieve or colander while you prep the remaining items to allow the cucumber to continue to drain.

2. When cucumber has totally drained, stir together all tzatziki ingredients. Season with additional salt, to taste.

Chicken:

1. Preheat oven to 400° F. Combine all herbs, spices, and salt in a small bowl. Brush both sides of chicken breasts with olive oil and sprinkle generously with

herb mixture. Bake until the meat thermometer reads 160° F, about 25-28 minutes for pretty thick breasts. Don't overcook! Remove from oven and set aside to fully cool.

Tabbouleh:
1. Combine all ingredients and season with additional salt, to taste.

Assemble Bowls:
1. Slice chicken breasts into about 1/2" slices against the grain. Divide slices equally among 5 meal prep containers. Divide tabbouleh and tzatziki equally among meal prep containers, as well. Spoon about 2-3 tablespoons hummus or baba ganoush into each container, to taste, and top with about 5 kalamata olives.

17. Chicken Sausage and Veggie Bake

Prep Time: 15 Minutes

Cook Time:30 Minutes

Total Time: 45 Minutes

Yield:: 4 Servings

Ingredients

- 1 package (4 links) cooked chicken sausage, sliced*
- 1 medium red onion, sliced
- 1 medium green bell pepper, sliced
- 1 medium red bell pepper, sliced
- 1 medium zucchini, halved lengthwise and sliced
- 1 cup chopped artichoke hearts (from a can)
- 2 tablespoons olive oil
- 1 ½ tablespoons honey
- ¼ teaspoon salt
- ¼ teaspoon red pepper flakes (or more to taste)
- ½ teaspoon dried oregano
- ¾ cup tomato sauce
- 1 cup shredded regular or dairy free mozzarella cheese
- ½ cup crumbled feta
- pita bread or naan, for serving

Instructions

2. Preheat the oven to 375°F.
3. Add the sausage, onion, both peppers, zucchini and artichoke to a 9 by 13 inch baking dish. Drizzle with the olive oil and honey, then sprinkle with the salt,

red pepper and oregano. Toss to combine and spread evenly in the dish.

4. Bake for about 20 minutes, stirring once halfway through, until the veggies are crisp tender.
5. Remove the dish from the oven and drizzle evenly with the tomato sauce. Sprinkle the top with the mozzarella and feta.
6. Return to the oven for about 10 minutes, until the cheese is nice and melted and the veggies are all tender.
7. Serve with the pita bread (or naan!).

18. Pickle-Brined Keto Fried Chicken

Prep Time: 10 minutes

 Cook Time:20 minutes

Total Time: 30 minutes

SERVINGS: 6

Ingredients

- 3 lb chicken thighs,, boneless and skinless
- 2 cups pickle juice,, from a jar of pickles
- 2 large eggs,, beaten
- 1 heaping tbsp mayo
- 1 tsp Dijon mustard
- 1/2 tsp coarse salt
- 1/4 tsp freshly ground black pepper
- 1-2 cup whey protein isolate, (or 1-2 cups finely crushed pork rinds)
- 2 cups avocado oil

Instructions

1. Place chicken in a large, resealable plastic bag. Pour pickle juice over chicken and place in refrigerator. Marinate for 8-24 hours, depending on how much pickle flavor you want your chicken to have (I go for the full 24)!

2. Drain chicken and discard pickle juice. Pat chicken
    dry and cut into 2-3 pieces each, if desired. Pat
    chicken dry with paper towels.

3. Mix together eggs, mayo, dijon, salt and pepper, then
    toss the chicken in the mixture, taking care to make
    sure it's entirely coated.

4. Preheat the oil in a large, deep skillet until
    shimmering. Working quickly, dredge each piece of
    chicken in whey protein (or pork rinds) and place in
    the oil. Cook until both sides are well-browned and
    chicken is cooked through, turning just once.

5. Drain cooked chicken pieces on paper towels. Serve
    with your favorite sauce. We like the Garlic Mustard
    Aioli from Trader Joe's (or make your own) or a
    good, homemade ranch dressing. Be happy that you
    can eat yummy things like this on a keto "diet"! :)

19. Sausage And Pepperoni Pizza-Stuffed Peppers

Prep Time: 25 minutes

Cook Time: 45 minutes

Total Time: 1 hour 10 minutes

Servings: 6

Ingredients

- 19.5 oz Italian sausage or turkey Italian sausage links, uncooked
- 1 T olive oil
- 1 small onion, chopped
- 1 T minced garlic
- 14 oz. jar pizza sauce (see notes)
- 2 tsp. dried oregano
- 3 large bell peppers, cut in half lengthwise and stem and seeds removed
- 3 oz. pepperoni
- 2 1/2 cups grated Mozzarella cheese

Instructions

1. Preheat oven to 375F/190C. Spray a 9" x 13" casserole dish or large baking sheet with non-stick spray or olive oil.

2. Heat olive oil in a large non-stick frying pan over medium-high heat and squeeze sausage out of the casings and add to the pan, breaking apart with your fingers as you add it. Cook until sausage is nicely browned, breaking apart with a turner or potato masher (affiliate link) as it cooks.

3. While the sausage cooks, cut 12 pepperoni slices in halves and the rest into fourths. Grate cheese if needed, or measure out desired amount of pre-grated cheese. Cut peppers in half and remove the seeds and cut out the stem end.

4. When sausage is nicely browned, push it to the side and add the onions and garlic. Turn heat to medium and cook onions and garlic 2-3 minutes.

5. Add the sauce and the dried oregano, turn heat to low, and simmer until the sauce is reduced and thickened. (You should be able to see the bottom of the pan if you pull your turner across it.)

6. Turn off heat, let the mixture cool for a few minutes, then add the chopped pepperoni and 2 cups grated Mozzarella, stirring gently so it's well-mixed with the sausage mixture.

7. Fill each pepper with the pizza-stuffing mixture, packing it in so all the stuffing is used. (It's easiest to hold the pepper in your hand over the pan while you fill and then add it to the baking dish.)

8. Bake peppers 20 minutes. Then remove from the oven and add a generous pinch of grated cheese and four pepperoni halves to the top of each pepper. Put back in the oven and bake 25 minutes more, or until the cheese is nicely browned, peppers are cooked, and the stuffing mixture is bubbling hot. Serve hot

20. Mexican Chicken Meal

Prep Time: 10 minutes

Cook Time: 12 minutes

Total Time: 22 minutes

Serving: 5

Ingredients

Southwestern Chicken
- 1 tablespoon garlic powder
- 2 teaspoons chili powder
- 1 teaspoon salt
- 1 teaspoon paprika
- 12 ounces boneless skinless chicken breasts 2 or 3 chicken breasts,
- 2 teaspoons avocado oil
- 2 teaspoons lime juice
- 1-2 cloves garlic peeled and smashed
- 1 avocado peeled and pitted
- 1 tbsp Freshly ground black pepper
- 1 tablespoon fresh lemon juice or lime juice
- 1 tablespoon white vinegar or apple cider vinegar plus more to taste
- 1/4 cup fresh parsley
- 1/3 cup fresh cilantro
- 1/2 teaspoon onion powder
- 1/2 teaspoon garlic powder
- 1/4 teaspoon paprika
- 3/4 cup unsweetened almond milk
- 1 teaspoon salt
- 10 eggs boiled to preference (see blog for recommendations)

- 12-15 snacking snacking peppers
- 2 1/2 cups mixed greens

Instructions

Cook Southwestern chicken:
1. In a small bowl, stir together garlic powder, chili powder, salt, and paprika. Reserve 2 teaspoons of seasoning and set aside. Evenly sprinkle seasoning over both sides of chicken breasts.
2. Heat avocado oil in a skillet over medium heat. When hot, gently add chicken breasts to skillet and sear on first side, about 5-6 minutes, or until it lifts easily. Flip and cook another 5-6 minutes, or until internal temperature reaches about 161-162° F. Drizzle with lime juice. Transfer to a plate and let rest at least 5 minutes.

Make avocado cilantro ranch dressing:
1. Combine all ingredients in a food processor or blender. Process until very smooth. Taste and add more vinegar, citrus juice, or salt to taste. Divide evenly among condiment cups or small reusable containers.

Assemble meal prep containers
1. Slice rested chicken breasts against the grain.
2. Evenly divide mixed greens among 5 meal prep containers. Evenly divide sliced chicken among containers and place on top of greens.
3. Evenly divide peppers among containers and place to the side of chicken and greens. Place 2 eggs in each container and sprinkle with reserved Southwestern seasoning. Serve with avocado cilantro ranch dressing.

DINNERS

21. Vegan Tortilla Soup

Prep Time: 20 minutes

Cook Time: 40 minutes

Total Time: 1 hrs

Servings: 6 people

Ingredients

- 2 tbsp olive oil
- 2 medium size shallots, peeled and chopped
- 1 lb peeled sweet potatoes, diced in 1/4 inch pieces
- 1 cup frozen corn
- 1 small jalapeno, seeds and ribs removed and finely chopped
- 3 large cloves garlic, peeled and minced
- 2 14.5oz cans black beans, drained
- 1 14.5oz can diced tomato
- 4 cups vegetable broth
- 1/4 cup chopped fresh cilantro
- 2 tsp ground cumin
- tsp ground chili powder
- 2 tbsp white vinegar
- kosher salt to taste
- corn chips or tortillas for topping

Instructions

1. In a large heavy bottomed pot or dutch oven, heat 2tbsp of olive oil over medium heat. Add the shallots, sweet potatoes, corn, and jalapeno and 1/2

tsp of kosher salt. Stir until the shallots and potatoes become softened, about 10 minutes.

2. Add the garlic, chili powder, and cumin and stir till fragrant. Then add your beans and tomatoes and stir to combine. Finally add your broth. Turn the heat up to medium high and allow it to come to a low simmer. Continue to simmer (not boil) for about 30 minutes.

3. Once the soup is ready, stir in any additional salt, 2 tbsp of vinegar, and fresh cilantro. Top with tortilla chips when ready to serve.

4. If you'd like to make your own tortilla chips like I did, preheat your oven to 400 degrees, brush your tortilla with olive oil on both sides, and bake for about 7-9 minutes until lightly browned.

Servings: 6

Ingredients

- 1 pound ground chicken
- 1-2 medium zucchini squash 1.5 cups shredded
- 2 garlic cloves, minced
- 2 tablespoons fresh chives, chopped
- 1/2 teaspoon kosher salt
- 1/4 teaspoon fresh black pepper
- 1-2 tablespoons oil for cooking
- Creamy Cilantro Sauce
- 1 cup fresh cilantro
- 1/2 garlic clove (or more depending on preference)
- 1/3 cup mayonnaise
- 1 tablespoon cottage cheese
- 1 tablespoon distilled white vinegar

Instructions

1. Combine cilantro, garlic clove, mayonnaise, cottage cheese, and vinegar in a food processor and blend till combined. Pop in the fridge to thicken and let flavors combine at least 30 min. You can also just chop the cilantro small and mix everything together by hand. Add salt and pepper to taste.

2. On a cheese grater, grate the fresh zucchini squash into small pieces and place on a paper towel. Sprinkle with a tiny bit of kosher salt and squeeze to remove excess moisture. Place into a large bowl

with chicken, garlic, chives, and 1/2 teaspoon kosher salt and a sprinkle of fresh black pepper. Form mixture into 3 inch patties, you should have 6 total.

3. Prepare a large nonstick or cast iron skillet with oil and bring to medium heat. Cook chicken patties on each side for 4 minutes until browned on both sides and cooked through. If they're not quite cooked through but getting really brown, pop them in the oven at 350 degrees for 2 minutes or so.

4. Serve warm with dipping sauce or top each popper with a little bit of the sauce.

23. TV Dinner Taco

Prep Time: 15 minutes
Cook Time: 22 minutes
Total Time: 42 minutes
Serves: 6-8

Ingredients

- Chimmichurri
- 2 cups cilantro
- 3 sprigs parsley
- 1 tsp oregano
- ½ cup red vinegar
- 8 cloves garlic
- 1 small lime wedge
- ¾ tsp red chili flakes
- 1 ½ tsp salt, to taste
- 1 tsp pepper to taste
- Garlic-Corn Mashed Potatoes
- 2 Russet potatoes, peeled and quartered
- 1 cup canned or fresh corn, pre-cooked
- 5 cloves garlic, minced
- 1 stick butter
- ⅓ cup heavy cream
- ¾ tsp each rosemary and parsley
- 1 tsp salt
- ¾ tsp pepper
- Ribeye
- 1 ½ lb(s) ribeye, thinly sliced

- 1 ½ Tbsp soy sauce
- ¾ tsp garlic powder
- ¾ tsp cumin
- ¾ tsp salt
- ½ tsp pepper
- ½ tsp sesame oil
- ½ tsp sugar
- butter
- Paratha
- 2 packs paratha (frozen)

Instructions

Chimmichurri

1. Pulse garlic with red vinegar in a food processor until finely chopped.
2. Combine cilantro, parsley, oregano, lime, red chili flakes, salt, and pepper with the chopped garlic. Pulse briefly until finely chopped.
3. Transfer to a bowl, and add the extra virgin olive oil. Adjust taste to your preference, and store in refrigerator until ready to serve.

1. Garlic-Corn Mashed Potatoes
1. Pre-cook the corn and set aside.
2. Bring a large pot of water to a boil. Add potatoes, boil until soft, approximately 20-25 minutes.

3. Drain, and place in a large mixing bowl. Heat butter in medium heat with garlic, rosemary and parsley for about 2 minutes. Then add the heavy cream and cook for another minute. Combine potatoes with the butter herb reduction.

4. Mix with an electric mixer or a potato masher to desired consistency. Salt and pepper to taste.

Ribeye

1. Combine beef with soy sauce, garlic powder, cumin, salt, pepper, sesame oil for a quick marinade.

2. Heat large pan in high heat. Lightly grease pan with butter. Make sure pan is very hot, and then add ribeye to the pan. Make sure to spread ribeye out evenly onto the pan for even cooking. Sprinkle the sugar on top, and let the beef char for a minute or two. Begin to stir fry until golden brown or desired level. Set aside.

Paratha

1. Keep paratha frozen until ready to cook. Heat medium size pan on medium heat. Place paratha on non-greased pan and cook for 1 minute, flip and continue until golden on both sides approximately 2-3 minutes. Ready to serve!

24. Roasted Chicken Dinner with Potatoes and Artichokes on a Bed of Crispy Kale

Prep Time: 10 minutes

Cook Time: 1 hour 10 minutes

Total Time: 1 hour 20 minutes

Severs: 4

Ingredients

- 4 skin-on, bone-in chicken drumsticks
- 4 skin-on, bone-in chicken thighs
- 1 whole skin-on, bone-in chicken breast, quartered (separate the breast and then cut each piece in half crosswise)
- EVOO, for drizzling
- Sea salt and freshly ground black pepper
- 1 ½ lb(s) baby potatoes
- 4 - 5 sprigs fresh rosemary, leaves stripped and chopped
- 2 small-to-medium onions, cut into thin wedges with the root ends attached
- 1 handful fresh bay leaves
- 1 frozen artichoke hearts, thawed, drained and halved, or 1 (14-oz) can artichoke hearts, drained and halved
- 1 head garlic, cloves separated and crushed
- 1 lemon, sliced

- 1 cup dry white wine
- 1 bunch black kale or dinosaur kale, stemmed
- Freshly grated nutmeg

Instructions

1. Drizzle the chicken with EVOO and liberally sprinkle with sea salt and pepper.
2. In a roasting pan or baking dish, combine the potatoes, rosemary, onions, bay leaves, artichokes, garlic and lemons. Drizzle with about 1/4 cup EVOO, season with salt and pepper and toss to coat. Arrange the chicken on top of the vegetables.
3. Position the rack on the center of the oven and preheat the oven to 350°F.
4. Roast the chicken and vegetables for 45 minutes. Turn on the broiler and douse the pan with the wine. Broil until crispy and brown, 12 to 15 minutes. Remove from the oven.
5. Dress the kale very lightly with about 1 tablespoon EVOO and season with salt, pepper and a few gratings of nutmeg. Spread the kale on a wire rack set over a baking sheet. Broil until very crispy, about 10 minutes.
6. Divide the kale among plates and top with the chicken and vegetables.

25. Roast Beef Dinner Salad with Cheddar

Serves: 4

Ingredients

Salad

- 10 cup (2.5 L) torn or baby Romaine lettuce
- 8 oz (250 g) thinly sliced roast beef, cut into strips (about 2 cups/500 ml)
- 1 cup (250 ml) chopped cooked or thawed green beans
- 1 cup (250 ml) crumbled Canadian old cheddar cheese
- 1 cup (250 ml) grape tomatoes, halved if large
- 1 cup croutons
- Dressing
- 1 cup (250 ml) milk
- ½ cup (125 ml) mayonnaise (light or regular)
- 2 Tbsp (30 ml) each, Dijon mustard and prepared horseradish
- ¼ tsp (1 ml) each, granulated sugar and dried thyme
- pinch Pinch each, salt and pepper
- ¼ cup (50 ml) red or white wine vinegar

Instruction

Salad

1. In a large bowl, toss lettuce with about 1/2 cup (125 ml) of the dressing to coat.

2. Divide among serving plates; top with roast beef, green beans, cheese and tomatoes. Drizzle with more dressing and sprinkle with croutons. (Any extra dressing can be covered and refrigerated for up to 3 days.)

Dressing

1. In a bowl, whisk together milk, mayonnaise, mustard, horseradish, sugar, thyme, salt and pepper; gradually whisk in vinegar.

2. Let stand for 5 min or until thickened

26. Chicken Tortilla Dump Dinner

Prep Time: 55 minutes

Cook Time: 1 hour

Total Time: 1 hour 55 minutes

Serves: 6-8

Ingredients

- 1 Tbsp canola oil
- 2 10-oz cans diced tomatoes with chiles, such as Rotel
- 1 cup chicken broth
- 1 Tbsp chili powder
- 1 Tbsp ground cumin
- ½ tsp kosher salt
- 1 15.5-oz can black beans, drained and rinsed
- 1 10-oz bag frozen corn
- 5 cups shredded cooked chicken (from about 1 small rotisserie chicken)
- 12 small corn tortillas, cut into quarters
- 1 8-oz block Monterey Jack cheese, shredded (about 2 cups)
- ½ cup sour cream
- ⅓ cup diced red onion
- ⅓ cup loosely packed fresh cilantro, chopped

Instructions

1. Preheat the oven to 375°F. Brush a 9-by-13-inch casserole dish with the oil.

2. Stir together the diced tomatoes with chiles, chicken broth, chili powder, cumin and salt in a large bowl. Add the black beans, frozen corn, chicken, tortilla wedges and half the cheese and stir to evenly distribute and moisten all of the ingredients. Transfer to the prepared casserole dish and spread into an even layer. Loosely cover with aluminum foil and bake for 25 minutes.

3. Raise the oven temperature to 400°F. Remove the foil and sprinkle the top with the remaining cheese. Continue to bake until the cheese is melted and just starting to brown, about 10 minutes. Top with dollops of sour cream and sprinkle with the red onion and cilantro. Serve hot.

27. Big Apple Salad

Prep Time: 30 minutes

Cook Time: 40 minutes

Total Time: 1 hour 10 minutes

Serves: 4

Ingredients

Spicy Walnuts

- 2 tsp (10 mL) kosher salt
- 2 tsp (10 mL) cinnamon
- 2 tsp (10 mL) ground ginger
- 2 tsp (10 mL) ground cumin
- 2 tsp (10 mL) chili powder
- 1 large egg white, whisked until foamy
- 2 cup (500 mL) walnut halves
- Apple Vinaigrette
- 2 Gravenstein apples, peeled, cored and finely diced
- 1 shallot, finely diced
- ½ cup (125 mL) fresh apple cider
- ½ cup (125 mL) canola oil
- 2 Tbsp (30 mL) apple cider vinegar
- salt and pepper
- Marinated Apple Rings
- 2 Gravenstein apples, cored and sliced into 1/8-inch thick rings
- ½ cup (125 mL) reserved Apple Vinaigrette

- 2 Tbsp (30 mL) thinly sliced flat leaf parsley leaves
- salt and pepper
- Blue Cheese Dressing
- ½ cup (125 mL) crumbled Danish blue cheese
- ¼ cup (60 mL) sour cream
- ¼ cup (60 mL) mayonnaise
- 2 Tbsp (30 mL) buttermilk
- 1 Tbsp (15 mL) apple cider vinegar
- salt and pepper

Salad

- 4 bunch watercress
- 1 Gravenstein apple, quartered, cored and thinly sliced
- 1 cup (250 mL) finely sliced celery hearts
- ½ cup (125 mL) chopped celery leaves
- ½ cup (125 mL) roughly chopped reserved Spicy Walnuts
- ½ cup (125 mL) sun-dried cranberries
- ½ cup (125 mL) Blue Cheese Dressing
- salt and pepper

Spicy Walnuts

1. In a small bowl, stir together salt, spices and egg white. Add walnuts and toss to coat evenly.

2. Spread walnuts in a single layer on a parchment paper-lined rimmed baking sheet and bake in a preheated 225 degrees Fahrenheit oven (110 degrees Celsius) until nuts are toasted and the coating is dry, about 1 hour, tossing every 20 minutes. Set aside.

Apple Vinaigrette

1. Combine apple, shallot, cider, oil and vinegar and season to taste with salt and pepper. Set aside.
2. Marinated Apple Rings
3. Toss together apple rings, vinaigrette and parsley, season to taste with salt and pepper, and let rest at room temperature until ready to serve.
4. Blue Cheese Dressing
5. Whisk together cheese, sour cream, mayonnaise, buttermilk and vinegar until smooth and season to taste with salt and pepper. Set aside.

Salad

1. Gently toss together watercress, apple, celery, celery leaves, walnuts and cranberries with dressing and season with salt and pepper to taste.
2. To Plate: Smear remaining blue cheese dressing on each of 4 chilled salad plates and mound salad on top. Place a stack of marinated apple rings on top of each salad, add a wedge of blue cheese and spoon over remaining apple vinaigrette. Serve immediately.

28. Barbecue Chicken and Brussels Sprout Sheet Pan

Prep Time: 10 minutes

Cook Time: 40 minutes

Total Time: 50 minutes

Severs: 2

Ingredients

- 4 bone-in, skin-on chicken thighs (1 1/2 to 2 lbs)
- 2 sweet potatoes, peeled and cut into 6 to 8 wedges each
- ¼ cup extra-virgin olive oil
- ¼ tsp chili powder
- Kosher salt and freshly ground black pepper
- ¾ lb(s) (about 3 cups) Brussels sprouts, halved and quartered depending on size
- ¼ cup barbecue sauce

Instructions

1. Preheat The Oven To 425°f And Line A Rimmed Baking Sheet With Parchment Paper. Place The Chicken Thighs Skin-Side Up On One Side Of The Baking Sheet, Spacing Them Evenly Apart. Roast Until They Turn Opaque On The Outside, 15 Minutes.
2. Remove The Baking Sheet From The Oven And Place The Sweet Potato Wedges In The Center. Drizzle The Potatoes With 2 Tablespoons Of The Olive Oil And

Sprinkle With Chili Powder And Some Salt. Use Tongs To Toss The Potatoes So Each Piece Is Evenly Coated. In The Remaining Open Area Of The Pan, Toss The Brussels Sprouts With The Remaining 2 Tablespoons Of Olive Oil And And Sprinkle With Salt And Pepper. Arrange The Brussels Sprouts Cut-Side Down On The Pan And Brush Each Chicken Thigh With Barbecue Sauce On All Sides.

3. Return The Baking Sheet To The Oven And Roast Until The Chicken Is Completely Cooked Through And Reads An Internal Temperature Of 160°f, And The Brussels Sprouts And Sweet Potato Wedges Are Tender And Charred In Spots, 25 To 30 Minutes More. Toss The Vegetables With The Accumulated Juices On The Tray Before Serving.

Prep Time: 20 minutes

Cook Time: 55 minutes

Total Time: 1 hour 15 minutes

Serves: 4

Ingredients

- 4 chicken legs, thighs and drumsticks separated
- Kosher salt and freshly ground black pepper
- 2 Tbsp vegetable oil
- ⅓ cup soy sauce
- ¼ cup sugar
- ¼ cup white distilled vinegar
- 5 cloves garlic, smashed
- 2 bay leaves
- 1 large yellow onion, sliced
- 2 scallions, sliced
- Cooked rice, for serving

Instructions

1. Season the chicken legs generously with salt and pepper. Turn the Instant Pot to the high saute setting. Add the oil and once it's shimmering, but not smoking, add half the chicken pieces and brown on

both sides, about 7 minutes. Remove with tongs to a plate and brown the remaining chicken pieces. Return all the chicken to the multi-cooker and add the soy sauce, sugar, vinegar, garlic, bay leaves, onion and 1/2 teaspoon pepper.

2. Follow the manufacturer's guide for locking the lid and preparing to cook. Set to pressure cook, on high, for 8 minutes. After the pressure cook cycle is complete follow the manufacturer's guide for quick release and wait until the quick release cycle is complete. Careful of any remaining steam, unlock and remove the lid and turn the Instant Pot back to the high saute setting. Let the sauce come to a boil and reduce it until dark brown and very fragrant, about 20 minutes. Remove the bay leaves.

3. Transfer the chicken and sauce to a serving platter, sprinkle with scallions and serve with rice.

30. Quick Taco-Style Chili

Prep Time: 45 minutes

Cook Time: 30 minutes

Total Time: 1 hour 15 minutes

Serves: 6

Ingredients

- 1 Tbsp neutral-flavored vegetable oil, such as canola or peanut
- 1 medium green bell pepper, stemmed, seeded, and chopped
- 1 medium white or yellow onion, chopped
- 2 large stalks celery, leaves discarded, chopped
- 1 clove garlic, finely chopped
- 1 lb(s) ground turkey or beef
- 1 pkg (1 oz) taco seasoning mix (see note below)
- 3 Tbsp tomato paste
- 1 can (14 1/2 oz) diced tomatoes with their juices
- 1 can (15 oz) pinto beans, drained and rinsed
- Salt and freshly ground black pepper
- Small cubes of avocado, for garnish
- Chopped fresh cilantro leaves, for garnish

Instructions

1. Press Sauté and select the middle temperature. Place the vegetable oil in the inner pot, wait about 1 minute

for the oil to warm, then add the bell pepper, onion, celery, and garlic. Cook with the lid off, stirring occasionally, until the onion softens slightly, about 5 minutes.

2. Add the turkey and cook, stirring occasionally to break it up into small pieces, until it is no longer pink, about 5 minutes.

3. Add the taco seasoning, tomato paste, and diced tomatoes, stirring to combine.

4. Close and lock the lid. Set the valve to Sealing. Press Cancel, then select High Pressure. Set the time to 20 minutes.

5. When the cooking cycle ends, carefully use a wooden spoon to release the pressure.

6. Press Cancel and remove the lid. Add the beans, stirring to distribute them evenly, then close and lock the lid to allow the residual heat to warm the beans, about 5 minutes.

7. Taste and adjust the seasoning, adding salt and pepper as needed. Serve the chili hot, garnished with the avocado and cilantro.

8. Quick Taco-Style Chili will keep, in an airtight container in the refrigerator, for up to 4 days.

9. More Flavoring and Serving Ideas for Quick Chili: